do you stutter:
a guide for teens

edited by
jane fraser
william h. perkins, ph.d.

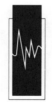

stuttering foundation of america
publication no. 21

First Printing — 1987
Second Printing — 1988
Third Printing — 1990
Fourth Printing — 1992

Stuttering Foundation of America
P.O. Box 11749
Memphis, Tennessee 38111-0749

Library of Congress Catalog Card Number 88-148588
ISBN 0-933388-27-6

The Stuttering Foundation of America is a non-profit charitable organization dedicated to the prevention and treatment of stuttering.

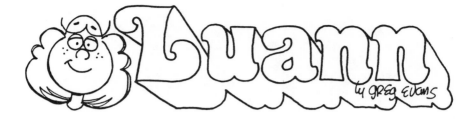

The Stuttering Foundation of America owes its thanks to Greg Evans, creator of LUANN cartoons, for sharing her with us. We feel that her presence has greatly enhanced this publication.

Thank you *GREG EVANS*

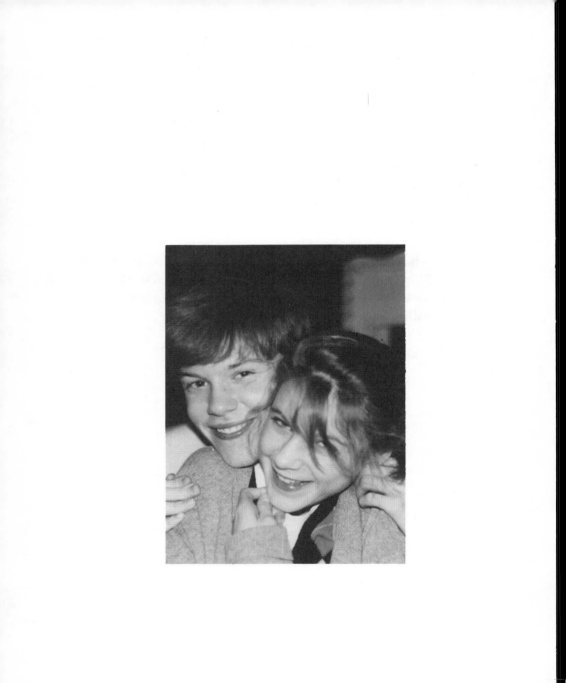

Foreword

Because you are a teen and because you sometimes stutter, some problems are uniquely yours. This book is written **to** and **for** you in the hope of helping you solve some of these problems.

Each chapter is written by a specialist in the field of stuttering. You may be interested to know that some of them have stuttered. Others have not. But all agree that much can be done to improve the quality of **your** life. We hope that this book will help you do just that.

Jane Fraser
President

Stuttering Foundation of America
September 1992

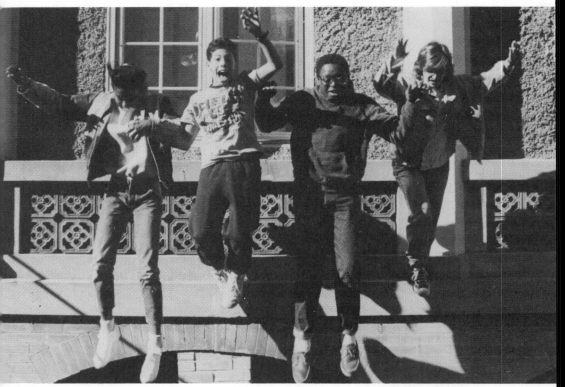

Photo Credit: Paul Diamond

Contents

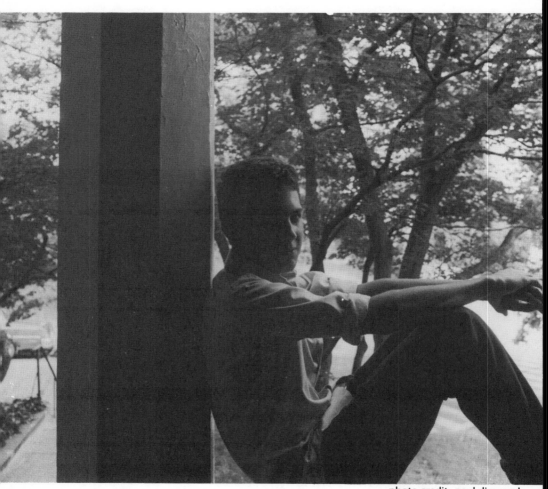

photo credit: paul diamond

Chapter
One

Why Me?

Richard F. Curlee, Ph.D.
Associate Dean of the Graduate College
University of Arizona

If you stutter, you have probably asked yourself thousands of times, why me?

All kinds of people stutter, prominent authors, actors, TV personalities, professional athletes, scholars, businessmen, even kings. Most, however, are just ordinary folks who are trying to get through school, or earn a living, or raise a family, or just be happy. Folks like you and me. At one time or another everyone in the world feels stupid, weak, worthless, ashamed, resentful, angry, fearful, or a little weird. If you stutter, however, it's tempting to believe that you feel this way *because* of stuttering. How about you? How do you feel about stuttering? How do you feel about yourself?

There is always some pain, some unhappiness in everyone's life. Some have more, some less. It's just a matter of degree. What does make a difference is what we do about what we don't like. What about you? Do you avoid calling people on the telephone? Do you substitute "easy" words for "hard" ones? Do you wind up feeling angry or frustrated trying to talk about something that's important? Do you keep quiet around strangers? Do you stay on the fringes at parties? Do you sometimes feel hopeless about improving your speech? You are not alone in these feelings, and this advice is written for you. You may not find all of the answers you are looking for, but you can gain a much better understanding of your stuttering and how to go about improving yourself by the time you finish.

Hiding

Most people try to hide things about themselves that they don't like. That's why millions of dollars worth of hair coloring, hair pieces, elevator shoes, make up, padded bras and the like are sold each year in this country. Sometimes, though, trying to hide makes things worse. It can even create worse problems than those you were trying to hide. If you find yourself avoiding speaking, or avoiding even participating in some activities, your world is revolving around stuttering. You are also acquiring some very costly lessons about stuttering and about hiding.

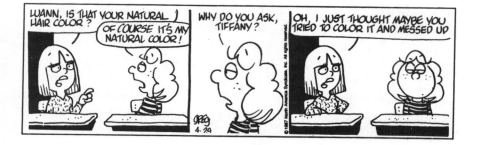

Fear almost always increases as a dreaded event gets closer and closer. Now, no one likes to feel scared, and all of us try to get rid of such feelings as quickly as possible. That's not always good, though. Because once we decide to avoid something because we might stutter, the relief that we feel "teaches" us to avoid similar situations in the future. In time, we usually find ourselves feeling increasingly scared about more and more situations. Do you spend a lot of time and energy worrying, plotting and planning how to keep from stuttering but little attention to changing when and how you speak? Does your world seem to be shrinking?

Avoiding speaking and avoiding stuttering are simply ways to hide. There are many others. Some try to camouflage anticipated difficulties by substituting words. Others say "uh" or "you know" to help get started or to postpone an anticipated block. Still others hold their breath, tense their jaw or blink their eyes to "help get the word out." Are any of these "tricks" familiar to you? Does stuttering seem like some sort of enemy, hiding inside, that you struggle and fight with on a daily basis? Is any of this really helping your speech? Are you feeling discouraged because previous efforts to improve your speech have failed? Are you afraid to give it another shot—afraid you will wind up feeling like a failure again? Read on.

Most of us try to avoid things that we dislike, and for those who stutter, that frequently means avoiding those situations or circumstances in which we are afraid that we will be embarrassed by stuttering. For example, do you often let others answer the phone even if you are closer? Do you sometimes order what you think you can say on a restaurant menu rather than what you want? Do you ever let teachers assume that you don't know an answer instead of responding in class? Do you wander around stores looking for what you want rather than asking where to find it? Do you find yourself agreeing with others because it might be difficult to express your disagreement? Is it your stuttering or the way people react that you hate most? Are you afraid just to be yourself? What, exactly, are *you* hiding from?

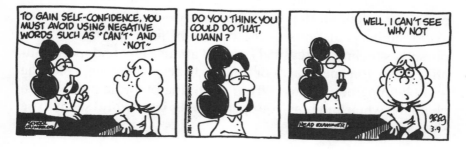

Self-Defeating Thoughts and Behavior

What you think affects what you do and how you feel. If you are like most folks who stutter, your stuttering comes and goes. You have good days and bad days. Sometimes you speak with scarcely any difficulty. At other times you could just die from the frustration and humiliation of stuttering. It's not unusual to hear guys who stutter say such things as:

> If I felt more secure, I wouldn't stutter.
> I just panic when that happens and my speech goes to hell.
> I stutter because I lack self-confidence.

All of this suggests that the way we feel dictates the way we speak. What do you tell yourself when you stutter? Have you ever thought that you must be stupid, or weak, or nervous, or whatever, because you stutter? Do such thoughts have anything to do with how you feel...with how you talk?

Listeners can be blamed for stuttering, too. For example, have you ever thought:

> I just can't keep from stuttering in front of strangers.
> Teachers blow my speech away.
> He seemed so busy and impatient that I just blocked.

These kinds of thoughts probably reflect, at least at first, feelings of helplessness that occur when we fail to achieve some goal we have. They are common to all of us, and in time, come to be believed. If you believe that you will fail if you try to walk a log across a creek, how does that affect the likelihood of your getting your feet wet if you try it? If you believe that you are going to stutter, how does that affect the way you speak? Does believing that your name is hard to say make it easier or harder to say? Does believing that you are just having a bad day make it easier or harder to work on your speech? Do you have any self-defeating beliefs? Are you ready to challenge your fears of speaking, your beliefs that you can not change your speech? Are you ready to get down to the nitty-gritty, the dirty work of changing? If so, you've come to the right book!

Taking Charge

Many people who stutter spend a lot of time trying to find out why they stutter. They believe that if they can get an answer to this question, they will be cured. Such beliefs, unfortunately, are not true and encourage people to focus on the past. Are you still spending a lot of time trying to find out why you stutter? Maybe it's time for you to start working on what you *can* change.

You already know the bad news—there's no known cure for stuttering. The good news is—you can change what you do. Feelings change when what we do changes. Our beliefs about ourselves change when our actions change. Sure, some changes are easy and some are not so easy. In fact, some changes may seem impossible at first. Perhaps this is how you feel now about your stuttering. Maybe you are down on your speech because previous efforts to improve were ineffective or short-lived. Maybe you even seemed to be "cured" for awhile until your speech relapsed. You would be crazy not to have doubts! It's one thing to talk, to hope for changes, but making those changes is not easy.

Talking is something you do. If you stutter when you talk, stuttering is something you do, too. With lots of work and effort on your part, and perhaps someone to help, you can stop avoiding those situations in which you fear you will stutter. You can stop trying to camouflage your stuttering. You can change how you talk. You can actually begin to free yourself from stuttering. But let's be clear on what that means. Almost always, recovery is a long, gradual process. There is no short cut, no easy way. You have to accept small steps in improvement. Substantial, lasting changes occur only over a long period of time. Unhappily, periodic relapses can occur, too. But even they can be overcome depending on how you respond. In the long run, however, you can stutter less, speak more comfortably and be less unhappy if you take charge of improving yourself. Is this an acceptable goal for you? Are you ready to assume responsibility for what you do? Is this the right time for you to take charge of how you talk?

Learning how to take charge of your life is part of growing up, an important part. But there is more to growing up than getting older, and there is more to taking charge than deciding what to do. You have to *do* what you decide. Now, there is every reason for you to doubt that it is possible to change something that seems so unchangeable at times. You may not even want to try to work on your stuttering right now. That's okay. There's nothing wrong with that. There can be many things in your life that are much more important than how fluently or disfluently you speak. If your stuttering is not bothering you now, there is no reason for you to go through the motions of changing it. Half-hearted efforts are doomed to fail, and trying to change just to please others has little chance of success. When you decide to work on your stuttering, it should be because you have made a commitment to yourself to change. It is something you have to do for yourself.

If you decide to read further, you will find out a lot more about stuttering and how you can go about getting help. This is the kind of book that has sections that you will probably want to reread several times. It may also raise some questions in your mind that you will want to think about for awhile. Perhaps you may even want to discuss some of them with a close friend or someone you trust, someone whose opinions you value.

Regardless of what you decide to do now, you should remember that many other folks out there are facing or have faced similar problems. Many probably had similar doubts and fears—and some of the hopes and dreams that you have, too. Not only are you not alone, there is understanding and assistance available to you. Well, that's it. No more questions. No more sermonizing. What you do next is up to you.

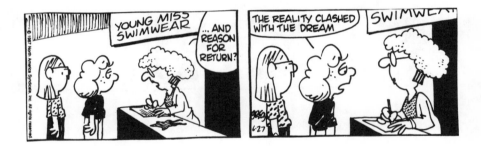

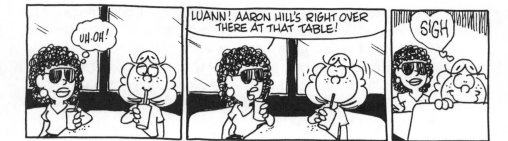

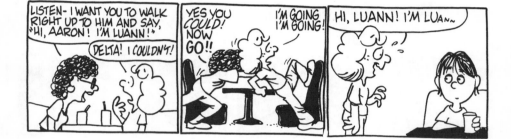

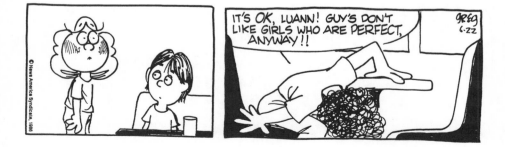

16

Chapter
Two

Facts and Myths

Edward G. Conture, Ph.D.
Professor, Department of
Communication Sciences and Disorders
Syracuse University

Once upon a time I was a teenager. So was your third period math teacher, your JV basketball coach and, believe it or not, even your mom and dad. Yeah, I know, those were the bad old days and things are much different now. And, I'd have to agree, some things like lasers, computers and the like are quite different today than when I was a teen. I think *you'd* agree, however, that some of these differences don't make much of a difference in terms of the way we think and feel about ourselves.

You May Be Unique but That Doesn't Make You Different

Think, for example, about that five-year old down the block learning to ride his first two-wheeler bike. Remember when you were first learning to ride your own two-wheeler? All those falls, the times you couldn't figure out how to stop the dumb thing and then when you finally rode it for more than 10 feet without falling? You might smile to yourself thinking about this little boy learning to ride his bike because it reminds you of your own experiences. What would happen, do you think, if you told this five-year old that you went through the same experiences yourself? Or, if you told him that you can remember how hard it was to learn to ride your bike and that is why he should do this or that to learn it easier and quicker? Chances are this five-year old might politely listen to your words of wisdom and then, shortly after you left, resume his own form of re-invention of the wheel!

You see, most of us—you, me and the little boy in our example—think of our experiences as unique, as a first time "thing." To a point, this is all right because each of us is unique. What we forget, however, is that even though we're each one of a kind, many of our experiences, like bike riding, are so similar that we can learn a lot from others who have previously had these experiences. Sure, each situation may be approached in a variety of ways but that's also okay. If we imagine, for example, a party where everybody is up dancing to the music, we would probably see that not everyone is dancing exactly the same way. What the dancers share with each other is the act of dancing to the music. They don't have to do exactly the same dance step to share the common experience of dancing. In other words, just because your particular approach to a situation is different, you'd be surprised to find how similar your reactions and feelings are to others experiencing the same situation. Yes, each of us is unique but that doesn't mean we are all that different from all others.

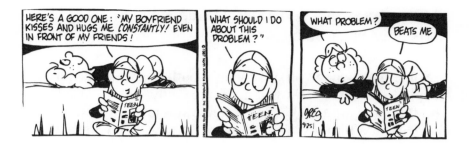

Most Problems are Similar, It's How We Handle Them That Differs

In fact, it's this similarity among peoples' problems that allows them to, for example, relate to the words of various popular songs. For instance, you may have never even heard of her, but it's pretty easy to understand Janis Joplin when she sings that sometimes "...it looks like everybody in this whole round world is down on me..." Or when Charlie Brown asks, "Why is everybody always picking on me." Sometimes, you too may feel a bit like Charlie Brown or the person in Joplin's song. Your problems seem to add up to the point where you think no one else could ever have such bad luck ("if it wasn't for bad luck, I'd have no luck at all"). However, the truth is that all people have problems. What *does* differ between people is the way in which they handle or cope with them. It's this coping skill, this ability to handle problems that really counts.

All of which leads me to the major point of my story. One good way for you to cope with your stuttering is to gain as much information as you can about your speaking problem. Now, I really can't tell you everything there is to know about stuttering but I can share with you some of our better, most current information about some aspects of stuttering that may be bothering you. This knowledge probably won't give you the power to "stop stuttering," but it will definitely help you see your problem a bit clearer which should help you to cope better.

"Stutterers Aren't Too Tightly Wrapped" and Other Fairy Tales

Sometimes when you open your mouth to speak it seems like people look at you as if you are not exactly with it. You know, you think they are looking at you like you are a little squirrelly, that's right, a bit nuts. Well, the first thing you should realize is that this is *their* problem, not *yours*. Our most current information suggests that stutterers, as a whole, are reasonably intact emotionally and psychologically. In fact, what amazes people who routinely work with stutterers, for example, speech-language pathologists, is that stutterers are so very normal given the fact that they frequently experience trouble talking. Of course, you are going to sometimes not want to talk when you actually know what to say. Other times you might avoid certain speaking situations but many times these fears of speech are, for the most part, normal reactions to abnormal events. I mean, wouldn't you think it a bit odd for someone to always enjoy doing something that was difficult for him to do. If you are in therapy, clinicians may try to help you minimize avoidances, fears and anxieties about speaking. They will understand that these are typical aspects of stuttering and not something to be ashamed of or hide. In any case, being a stutterer and having these concerns in no way means you are crazy, nuts or off balance. You are merely reacting in ways that are normal under the circumstances.

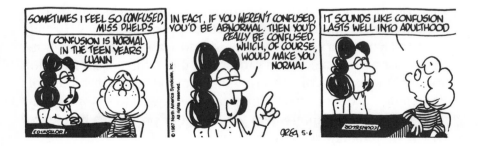

20

Listeners May Be the Ones Who Actually Get Nervous in the Service of Talking

One of the more common sayings about stutterers, which I'm sure you've heard, is that "...they stutter because they are nervous." However, what is never asked is whether the listener who says that you are nervous was also nervous! Many times people attribute feelings to others that they themselves have. For example, a listener who just can't stand to wait for anything (like a traffic light) may get "nervous" waiting for stutterers to finish their thoughts. A listener who feels nervous when you stutter may assume that you share these feelings and that these feelings are the root cause of your speaking problems. Hence, it is no wonder that so many listeners—all well intentioned, of course—frequently tell you to "relax."

Of course, it's difficult for anyone to speak clearly and fluently when they are tense. On the other hand, too much relaxation leads to sleep, not fluency! You, me and everybody must have a reasonable balance between tension and relaxation to speak at our best. We don't want to be so tense as to imitate the Tinwoodsman from the Wizard of Oz nor so relaxed as to be like the Scarecrow either. We're probably more like Gumby with some degree of tension and relaxation thrown in together. Anything which upsets the balance between tension and relaxation makes it difficult for any of us to speak as smoothly as possible.

Question: How Do You Get a One-Armed Stutterer Out of a Tree?
Answer: You Wave at Him

Some people think that *anybody* who is slightly different from normal is generally not very bright. Unfortunately these same people don't like to have any information cloud their judgments and opinions. If anything, existing information strongly suggests that most stutterers are well within the normal range of intelligence. Stutterers go to college and hold various responsible positions in a variety of professions. Actually, the old idea some people may have that stutterers aren't as smart as the next person is just another version of "stutterers are nervous." Humans many times blame one problem, in this case stuttering, on another problem, in this case intelligence, regardless of whether there is another problem in existence at all! As far as we can tell, stutterers have just as much right to be a genius as anyone else. In short, normally fluent people don't have a lock on intelligence! No, the chances are very good that you weren't standing in the wrong line when they were handing out the brains.

You Can Take the Stuttering Out of the Stutterer But You Can't Take the Stutterer Out of the Stutterer

While it is true that some stutterers continue to stutter for long periods of time, many change their speech and walk away from their problem with only occasional looks backward. Sure, it takes courage, work and patience to change something as personal as your speech—we never said any of this was going to be easy—but change it you can! Our best, most current information indicates that your behavior isn't poured into a mold like so much concrete. It's changeable; however, it's really up to you to do the changing. Of course, to make some of these changes you'll have to have a "little help from your friends," like a speech-language pathologist. Time after time, stutterers have shown themselves and those around them that they can change, that they can become increasingly more fluent. They don't have to do what they do and remain who they are if they don't really want to.

Stuttering is Learned by Imitation or Parrots Can Talk but Can They Order from the Menu

We've never heard of one crow, mynah bird or parrot—all famous imitators—who began to stutter through living with and imitating a stutterer! Furthermore, normally fluent speech-language pathologists who have worked with literally hundreds of stutterers haven't—through all their exposure to stuttering—either "picked-up" or come to imitate the problem. Most stutterers began stuttering without ever having heard anyone also stutter. However, the imitation myth dies hard, so too did the one about warts on your hands from handling frogs and toads. In part, the imitation myth's refusal to die relates to our belief that children copy the habits of their elders like so many little copy machines. While this copying may be at least partially true for certain behaviors, it's hard to figure how this works with stuttering when the child's elders, for example, parents, seldom stutter. No, stuttering doesn't seem to be something that spreads like a cold or enters the body like radioactivity. In theory, a parrot should be able to imitate a person stuttering but we know of no such case. It's our best guess, based on current understanding of speech and related events, that imitation is an overly simplistic explanation for the cause of an extremely complex problem.

You Got Your Green Eyes From Your Mom and Your Stuttering From…

Stuttering seems to run in some families. Does this mean that stuttering is inherited? No one really knows for sure. Some scientists have found what seems to be a genetic basis for certain speech and language difficulties which may eventually result in stuttering. However, if inheritance is a factor in stuttering, its role is quite complex and not as predictable as the inheritance of eye or hair color. Furthermore, for many stutterers, it would seem that this inheritance factor plays a less important role.

Stress May Fracture Your Bones But How About Your Speech?

If anyone had reason to stutter because of stress, then the air traffic controllers at our major airports should have reason. However, there has not been a break-out of stuttering in the air traffic control towers, at least not that we know of! No, stress doesn't help anyone do anything at their best but, like death and taxes, stress is a fact of life. To think that one can lead a life free of stress is a little bit like waiting up all night to get the tooth fairy's autograph. Both events will never come to pass.

Life is full of events that stress us in mental, psychological and physical ways. Indeed, it is often from these stressful events that we learn the most about ourselves, for example, good feelings about yourself when successfully finishing a difficult book report for English class. Obviously, constant, unrelieved stress is no good for anyone but neither is trying to walk through life in a dream-like state. Whatever we believe that stuttering is, it is not "caused" by stress anymore than saying that salt rubbed into a knife wound "caused" the wound. Rather, it's the knife that caused the cut in the first place and the salt only makes the wound hurt. Unfortunately, just like in an unsolved murder mystery, we still haven't found the knife that causes stuttering but we are fairly sure that stress is sometimes the salt that makes the problem worse.

Nothing Goes Better with Fatigue, Not Even Speech

Although various situations are frequently associated with stuttering, three of the more common ones are: talking during excitement, rapid talking, and talking when overly fatigued. At the end of a hard day of school, work or sports not even Abraham Lincoln would like to deliver the Gettysburg Address! When people are mentally, emotionally and physically tired, it is just not as easy for them to maintain fluent speech. When people are overly tired they can't dance as well, compute the latest national debt figures or paint within the lines. Simply put, fatigue makes it more difficult for a person to maintain fluent speech, to perform at his or her best in general. However, fatigue is a bit like stress, it can be minimized but it can't be totally avoided. It might help to realize that most people find that fluency just can't be as easily maintained during certain emotional/physical states and leave it at that. Trying to avoid being fatigued is a bit like trying to avoid getting nervous or stop thinking about pink elephants! In fact, one can get pretty fatigued trying not to get fatigued as well as pretty nervous trying not be nervous!

Stuttering Severity Fluctuates or the Pendulum Never Stops in the Middle

It is said that one thing is constant and that is change. Your weight, the weather, your school grades and your stuttering all fluctuate (not to the same degree, we hope)! What probably makes these swings in your stuttering so puzzling to you is the same thing that puzzled early humans about the weather: its seeming unpredictability. You are fluent one moment and stuttering the next. While your instances of stuttering are not quite like an earthquake whose violent, unpredictable comings and goings threaten our very lives, the seeming randomness of your stuttering may remind you of the sudden, unexplained eruptions of a volcano. Here one day, gone the next.

While no one knows precisely why stuttering fluctuates the way it does, it most probably relates to changes in: your reactions to listeners and situations, the complexity of the speaking situation, how fast you talk, and so forth. Perhaps even changes in fatigue and stress may play a role as well but whatever the case, it's fair to say that change in your stuttering is fairly constant! This change, we know, can be discouraging but at least you should know that it is a typical part of the stuttering problem of most stutterers.

More Men Stutter than Women Or Where Was the Equal Rights Amendment When You Really Needed It?

At present, it is estimated that there are two million stutterers in the United States. It's also a fact that three to four boys stutter for every girl who stutters. To begin, let me say that we don't know the *exact* reason for this difference between men and women. However, besides a handful of exceptions, men exhibit more of just about every human problem than women. Is this fair? No, of course not, but it's a fact of life. There are far more men in prison than women, younger men have far more car accidents than women, and so forth. Why this difference? First, during early childhood development, there are innate differences between boys' and girls' speech and language abilities. Second, during this same period, the home as well as social environment appears to react to boys somewhat differently than girls. Therefore, more boys stutter than girls probably because of inherent differences in boys' speech and language abilities *and* differences in the environment's reactions to the boy's abilities and behavior.

In truth, all these differences really make little difference to you. What is important, and what you should try to remember, is the fact that just because you are a boy doesn't mean you *have* to stutter the rest of your life.

In other places in this book you'll find some suggestions of how you can go about changing your speech and related behavior for the better. These suggestions, just like the "facts" I've discussed with you, represent our attempts to speak the truth to you. And, to paraphrase an old saying, we hope these truths will start to help set you free of your problems.

That's the facts, Jack.

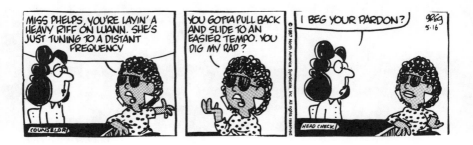

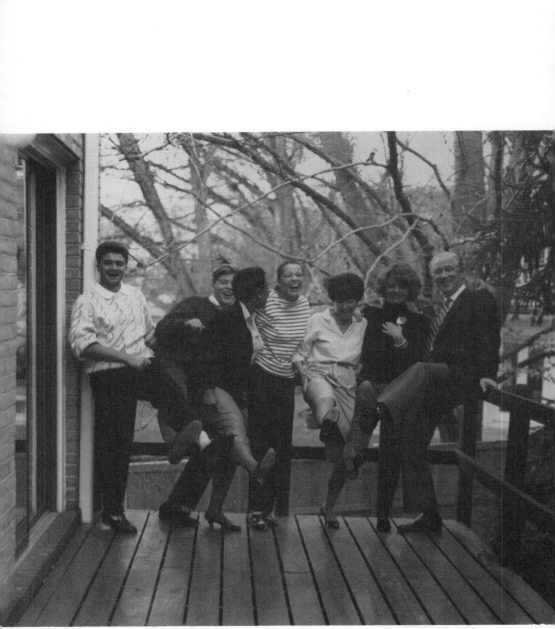

photo credit: celia gruss

28

Chapter
Three

Coping With Parents

Dean E. Williams, Ph.D.
Professor Emeritus
Department of Speech Pathology and Audiology
University of Iowa

Stuttering can create a different kind of problem between you and your parents than most any other one that you're apt to run into.

As you've grown up, your parents have told what you what to do and not do, how to behave and not behave, what to eat and not eat, and so forth and so forth and so forth. You've argued about some things, agreed with some others–you did some of the things they suggested, didn't do others–told your parents what you've done at times and not told them at other times. Issues or problems between you and your parents often are out in the open where you can talk about them, laugh at them, cry because of them, argue and even yell about them. But, at least most of the time you talk to each other. For most teenagers, the problems of stuttering aren't like that.

When you talk with your parents, you're apt to be spending much of the time while you talk in trying as hard as you can to hide your stuttering and they spend most of their time pretending not to notice when you do stutter. You're both–in varying degrees–uncomfortable and yet it seems to be something that you and your folks pretend not to notice–and as a result, don't talk about. This leaves you feeling rather sad–and worried. And, people who care about each other do worry. They worry about what the other is thinking and feeling. When they don't talk about it, they have to imagine what the other thinks. When you *imagine* what your folks think about your stuttering, you, like everyone else, imagine the worst. Stuttering is *awful* to you, therefore, your parents must be thinking *"awful"* things about it and–possibly–even about you. Add to this the fact that at times they do such things as finish words for you, talk for you, look away from you when you begin to stutter, or tell you to "take your time," or "think what you want to say," among other things. When your parents do and say things like that it doesn't help, it only adds to your worry–and to your feelings of being all alone–and not knowing what you can do about it.

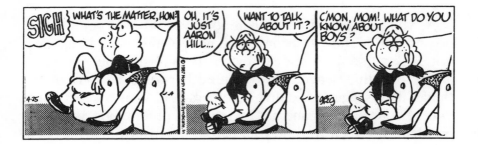

30

I want to discuss with you problems I have found that teenagers and their parents often have in facing the stuttering problem openly. I hope that you will find that some of the questions I ask are those that you have thought of and have worried about.

Do Your Parents Act Like Stuttering Is Something They Don't Want to Talk About?

If you think that your parents do that, you aren't alone. It's one of the most common concerns I hear from teenagers. You might be surprised at some of the responses parents give.

One reason for not wanting to talk about it is that they are afraid it would upset their child if they showed disappointment in the ways the child talks. They go on to say that their child doesn't talk to them about it and appears to be upset and embarrassed when stuttering occurs. This makes them feel that it is a very private and personal thing to their child–and they respect this and don't want to intrude. Isn't this interesting? *You* don't talk to them because you believe *they* don't want to talk about it and *they* don't want to talk to you because they believe that *you* don't want to talk about it! This may seem like an odd situation and yet it is not unusual at all. Let me take an example that does not involve speech. If a good friend of yours does something during class in school that is embarrassing, you are likely also to feel embarrassed for your friend. If you like this person, you are apt to not talk about it after class–not because you thought what was done was so *awful* but because you respected your friend's feelings.

31

You see, this is what some–perhaps your–parents do too. They do it *not* necessarily because you *stuttered* but because they can see that you are upset by it–and they respect your feelings.

Another reason that some parents give me for not talking with their child about stuttering is that it is no big issue with them. It doesn't bother them too much–they've gotten used to it. In fact, they may state something to the effect that "we only came today to find out about it because we were told that we should."

These parents may tell me that their child doesn't stutter too much around them. He's one who doesn't have much to say about things. He likes to be alone a lot so he can read, and listen to his music. "He's our quiet one." He's not like his younger brother who "talks all the time and is very out-going."

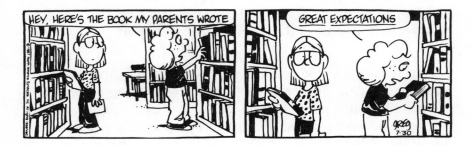

There is no way for them to know that you are avoiding situations where you would have to speak–not because you like being alone but because you're afraid you will stutter. They can't see the times you substitute words, or the times you just nod your head instead of speaking, or the times you talk only when you think you can say it without stuttering. They don't know how you feel inside **unless you tell them.**

A third, and the most common reason that parents give me for not talking to their teenager about stuttering is that they just don't know very much about it and they don't know what to say about it. They feel badly about this. They have helped their child grow up to where today they have an ever increasingly independent teenager. Over the years they were able to understand your fun times, your problems, your successes and your failures–because they had experienced them as they grew up. They are able to help and guide you from their own experiences–Oh, you argue and you may yell at each other some–but still you both generally know where each is coming from–you just don't agree, that's all. And, that's alright. Most of the time you've worked it out–or agreed not to work it out–because it was out in the open where you both could talk about it. But, stuttering isn't like that. Your parents may not be stutterers. They don't know what it's like. Yet, as your parents, they believe that they should know how to help.

Now, if you will, try to "walk in their moccasins" as an Indian was once supposed to have said. They don't know what to say or to do to be helpful. They don't understand–and they feel somewhat embarrassed and even helpless because they don't. They may bluster at times and tell you to do this or to do that with the hope that it might help. But, mostly that's what it is–a hope–that it might help. The fact that, in most instances, it doesn't help much only makes them feel badly–and, you sad, or, even angry. Can you begin to see how important it is that you and your parents talk? There reaches a point where one must quit pretending that the stuttering problem can be hidden. You're unhappy because you stutter. Your parents are unhappy because they don't know what to do or say to be helpful. It's time to talk with each other.

Most of the time in the past when you and parents talked about a problem, it was your parents who started the conversation. In this instance however, your stuttering is your problem and it is up to you to begin the conversation. For some of you, this will not be too difficult. Your parents are fairly open and easy to talk to about problems that concern you. For others of you who have not talked to your parents much about any of your problems, it can be tough. From my experience of talking to many teenagers about this problem, I find that the *toughest* part for them is to summon up the courage to begin the conversation. You may think that you don't have the courage, but I'll bet you do.

All of the teenagers I've talked to have considerable courage. Too often they doubt their courage because of the times they reported that they didn't have "the nerve to talk," because they were afraid they would stutter. I always respond to this by asking them to tell me the times in the last two or three days when they have talked even though they felt that they would stutter. If they did this even once–and all of them had–it took courage on their part.

You most certainly have talked at times when you felt scared inside. You were fairly certain that you would have trouble speaking but you spoke anyway. This took courage.

You should expect to feel uncomfortable, *a little scared,* when you begin to talk to your folks about a problem that is as personal as your stuttering is to you. I want to make some suggestions that should help make it easier. Teenagers have told me that they help. They're worth a try.

First, select a good time and place to talk. Many families seem always to be in a hurry–Mom and Dad often are hurrying after getting home or are hurrying to go some place or are hurrying so they can hurry to do something else. And, don't overlook the fact that often you are doing the same thing. Therefore, **find** a time when there is **time** to talk. Examples of such times include when you're riding together in a car or when you're sitting around the table after dinner. Most families have times when it's easier to talk with each other. Look for them. It can be with just one parent if that is more comfortable. Many report that it's easier to talk when you're doing things together–and when no one else is around.

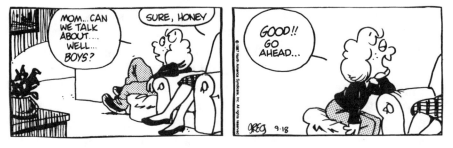

Second, be aware that your parents are likely to feel awkward too. They may look down and fidget or sound rather abrupt or even act a little embarrassed. Don't let these kinds of reactions get to you. Just remember that your folks have feelings too and–just like you–there are times when, at first, they don't know what to say. For example, have you figured out yet how to talk to them about sex and have them look you in the eye as they answer–and not blush?

Third, think about the above two points I've just discussed. I hope that you now can see how important it is that *you* start the conversation and set the tone for it. Be straightforward and direct in what you say. It can help if, at the same time, you acknowledge your own discomfort. Some examples include: "I want to talk to you about my stuttering." Then continue with, "I don't know exactly how to begin," or, "I'm embarrassed by it," or "it's hard to talk about" or any other statement that reflects the way you feel at the time. Now, you've taken the first big step! You're free to follow-up with any issue that you want to talk about. You don't have to talk about all of them at one time. Pick several that are especially important to you and begin with them. The door is now open to talk about your stuttering at other times, in other places–and remember–you will need to do your share to keep the door open. Here are some issues that are likely to come up.

Do Your Parents Finish Words for You and At Times, Talk for You?

If you are like most teenagers, your parents do this, or have done it. Parents report to me that they are only trying to help their child. You can explain to them that it really doesn't help. If you are afraid that they will finish words or will talk for you, you have more trouble than you would otherwise. Explain to them that it is important to you that you do your own talking–that they will help the most by waiting for you to say what you want to say. Once again look at it for a moment from their standpoint. If, when you begin to stutter, they finish the word for you and you then quit trying and just nod in agreement, it looks to them as if they have helped. If, on the other hand when they finish your word, you don't stop but continue to stutter until you finish it, it is obvious to them that they are not helping. The same thing is true when they talk for you. If you quit talking and nod in agreement, it looks to them as if they are helping. But, if you continue to talk– even though you stutter–and say what you want to say (even though it may be what your parents just said) it becomes obvious to them that they aren't helping. In this way you show them that you can do your own talking.

Do Your Parents Think That If You Really Tried You Could Stop Your Stuttering?

Regardless of what they think, you know that it isn't true–and you are right. You know that when you try as hard as you can, when you do everything you can figure out or that people tell you will help, you stutter anyway. Often you stutter more. Your parents need to understand this about stuttering. Explain to them about the ways you feel and the things you do to try to help. If they can't understand it from you, then they need to talk to a speech-language pathologist.

Do Your Parents Make Special Allowances For You Because You Stutter?

There are times when your parents may excuse you from doing certain jobs around the house that involve speaking, for example, running errands. You know that at first you feel relieved–but you're embarrassed too. And, you're not too proud of yourself if you know that a friend or your brother or sister do jobs like these. Here is a very important reason to be able to talk to your folks. Explain to them that you may be scared at times but that you want to do your share. You'll feel better and they will too–and it will be one more step in helping them understand your stuttering problem. You will need to be alert thereafter and be ready to volunteer to help around the house, run errands, or anything else where some talking may be necessary.

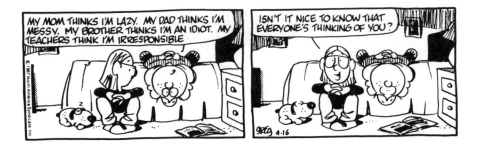

Do Your Parents Seem To Be Irritated or Angry at Times Because You Stutter?

This is a tough question to consider because it is necessary to separate the ways you act when you are actually stuttering from the ways you act either because you are afraid that you will stutter, or because you have just stuttered. Parents tell me that they aren't angry or irritated *when* their child stutters. But, they go on to tell me that they will become angry when he or she is rude or sullen or thoughtless of others. The examples they give include such things as "when Bert answers the phone, he stutters, and hangs up. He didn't know who was calling, the purpose of it, or anything else. He just hung up. He was rude and thoughtless." Another example was when "some friends stopped by to see Marcia. They were talking and having fun. They suggested to her that they go after a pizza and meet some boys. She then became sullen and rude. She had been stuttering some. She quit talking and told them that she was not going to go along."

The above examples should be enough to make the point. You may act at times in ways that aren't polite or friendly *because* you very much do not want to stutter. Your parents don't understand this and therefore are likely to say something to you about being impolite and rude. Down deep, you don't like yourself for the ways you acted—but the fact that your parents jump on you about it only makes it worse. This is one more reason that you and your parents need to talk so that you can help them understand stuttering—so to speak—from the horse's mouth.

Do Your Parents and You Disagree About the Need for Therapy?

There are instances when parents push their teenagers to receive therapy and they are reluctant to do so. There are others where teenagers want therapy but the parents think it is not necessary. Do you fit into either of these categories? If so, I hope that it now is obvious that you and your parents need to talk. You both need to discuss—openly—the reasons "for" and "against" receiving therapy. It usually isn't a difficult decision to make if it is based on a mutual understanding. If it can't be made this way, I always recommend that you and your parents discuss it with a speech-language pathologist. If one isn't available, then why don't you speak with a counselor or teacher at school? They are not emotionally involved and can be helpful.

A Closing Thought

A good way for you to cope with your parents and for them to cope with you and for you both to learn to cope with stuttering is for you to ask them to sit down and read this chapter. Then you can sit down together and discuss the parts that apply to you and to them. Just by discussing it together will build a foundation for constructive coping–and the basic elements of helpfulness for both of you.

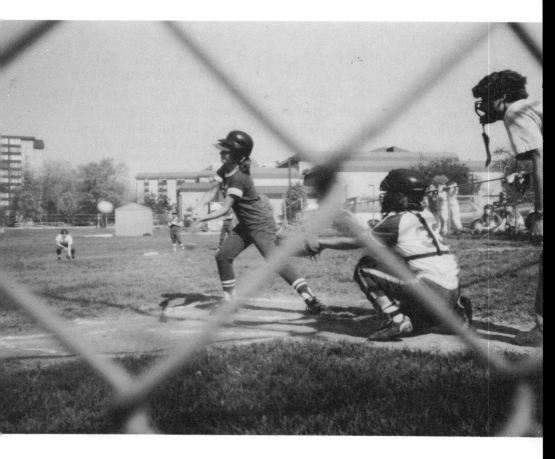

Chapter
Four

Coping With School

Hugo H. Gregory, Ph.D.
Director of Stuttering Programs
Professor and Head
Speech and Language Pathology Program
Northwestern University

Coping with your stuttering in the school environment is doubly important because you spend so much of your time there and because talking in school is vital to your success as a student. The kind of impression you feel that you are making contributes to the feelings you have about yourself. Participating in class activities, interacting with fellow students and teachers, and therapy as related to school activities, are topics teenagers who stutter say that they think about a great deal.

Reciting in Class

Almost all who stutter have experienced the frustration of saying, "I don't know," when they did know, rather than take the chance of stuttering as they answered a question in class. At that moment, fear of stuttering is relieved, but later you feel frustrated because you are not demonstrating your true potential.

Students who stutter always refer to the anticipation of what they call "reading up and down the rows." Nonstuttering students scan ahead to see if there are words they don't know or can't pronounce. **You** scan ahead in a reading passage to see if there are words you may stutter on in the section you anticipate reading when it is your turn. But, not only are you fearing being blocked, a very threatening experience; you may also be wondering if a student will laugh. You may dislike the possibility that students are uncomfortable when you speak. As a result of previous difficulty and these reactions, you experience more fear and tension.

Giving reports is another commonly feared situation, although some students do better when they get up before the class and know that they have full attention. Some find that practicing a report many times alone makes it easier when giving the report in class. You might want to ask the teacher to give you more time during class discussion if you have found it easier when you take your time. Time pressure–your feeling that you must not keep your listener waiting and that you may not be able to start talking again if you pause–may cause you to speak more rapidly and be afraid to pause. By not hurrying, you reduce this time pressure. Although it is hard to participate in class discussion and answer questions when you anticipate stuttering, avoiding such situations appears to increase tension and stuttering. One junior high school girl who had made much improvement in her speech experienced insecurity about entering high school. She told her teachers that she would be more comfortable if not called upon to recite in class. After a few weeks of being excused from participating in speaking situations, her fear of speaking was greater and her speech became much worse.

Going ahead in spite of trouble usually makes one feel better–and is better for you! However, avoiding and not talking or being willing to speak even though you stutter are both difficult.

Getting therapy in which you are learning to modify your speech, deal with time pressure, and decrease your stuttering in situations varying systematically from easier to more difficult, is the most positive and the most hopeful way of improving your participation in school activities. You and the speech pathologist can plan with your teacher the ways in which you are going to work the procedures you are learning in therapy into your talking in the classroom.

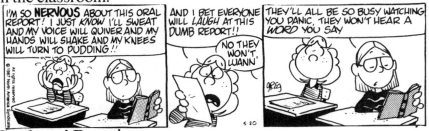

Students' Reactions

"A lot of kids feel bad about themselves, so they try to make others feel bad."

"People try to find things that are wrong with others. Stuttering is very obvious."

These statements by two junior high school students who are in therapy reflect a way in which many students interpret negative reactions to their stuttering. In teen years students move rapidly from childhood feelings and behavior into the pressure and demands of adulthood. There is much mixed emotion. Students try to build themselves up by cutting others down. Psychologists believe this reaction is the basis for much of the prejudice that exists today. Students who stutter have admitted that they have made fun of fellow students who are, for example, overweight. Then it dawns on them that they are doing the very thing they believe others should not do to them. People who make fun of others are expressing their own inadequacy even if they don't intend to hurt.

You can help your fellow students by being more open about your stuttering. This may be hard if you believe that by not thinking and not talking about it, the stuttering will disappear. If you have reached your age and still have a problem, it may be time to be more realistic and open about it. Talk to friends. Talk to your teachers. And even talk to those who hassle you. Nothing stops them like saying, "Yes, I have a stuttering problem," or "I sometimes stutter and I'm working on it."

A girl stutterer, age 16, commented, "Kids get less mean as times goes on. But, you don't have to wait it out. Give them some help." A fourteen year old boy just beginning therapy, told me that he was taking more responsibility now for helping his friends at school feel more comfortable about his stuttering. He tells them about therapy and mentions his difficulty from time to time when he stutters. For example, he may say, "I really hit that sound hard. I can do it easier."

Teens tell me of being surprised to find that many people want to learn more about stuttering. For example, they may be very pleased by the interest shown when they make a classroom speech about stuttering. Of course, it is probably easier to be more open about your stuttering if you are receiving therapy and have greater hope of improvement.

The Teachers' Reactions

Just as you like certain teachers better than others, you will or will not like the way some teachers react to you and your stuttering. From group session, I have found some teenagers prefer that

44

teachers never say anything about their speech problem. Others appreciate their teachers' interest and concern. One student said, "It irritated me that the teacher was giving me special attention." Another said that she appreciated the teacher asking her after school, "Is there some way in which I can help?"

How can we explain these differences? If you and your family have participated in "a conspiracy of silence" about your stuttering at home, then you may have adopted a policy of not talking about your speech and not wanting anyone at school to mention it. This attitude of going it alone can be tough! Three teenage stutterers agreed in talking with me recently that it is better to talk with teachers about your problem "if it can be done in an intelligent way." By "intelligent" they meant that teachers talk with them about their feelings and what they think could help them to participate more successfully in class. If they were receiving therapy, they wanted the speech pathologist and the teacher to include them in discussions—not to talk behind their backs. There are differences in the ways teachers relate to a sensitive matter, but sometimes your own sensitivity may hamper a teacher's efforts.

Some teachers, perhaps due to a lack of experience with students who stutter, may be puzzled and uncomfortable when you stutter. They may be embarrassed. Talking with such teachers may help them to deal with their own feelings and to be more comfortable.

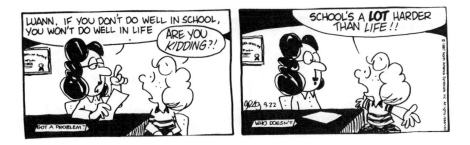

The School Situation and Stuttering Therapy

Some students who stutter don't want it known that they are in speech therapy, and others simply refuse to have therapy in school. You should not feel guilty about this because it results in part from the ways in which people have reacted to you and your stuttering problem. You have a right to be embarrassed! Later, as your speech is improving in therapy, as you are feeling less alone in coping with your difficulty, and as you are becoming less sensitive, you may be more willing for others to know that you are working on your speech.

As you improve, you and your speech pathologist can use the school to work on your speech in settings of varying difficulty. In this connection, you may wish to talk to your teachers about your therapy goals–either alone or with your clinician. Most teens I've worked with have been willing to show what they are doing in therapy to their friends. Oftentimes, when audio and video recordings are made, the student in therapy realizes how much better his good speech skills are compared to those of the friend. This is very rewarding! Speaking better often sounds and feels strange at first and you are hesitant to think that your friends will notice you are different. However, you are more likely to be aware of changes in your speech than anyone else. Therapy helps you accept the change involved in speaking better.

By establishing realistic goals and taking responsibility, you can speak better and better and feel more and more comfortable about it.

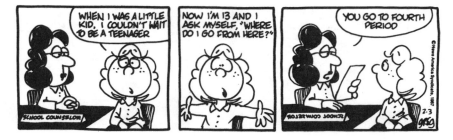

Chapter Five

Coping With Friends

Lois A. Nelson, Ph.D.
Professor
Department of Communicative Disorders
University of Wisconsin-Madison

Do You Wish You Had Friends You Could Really Talk To?

Friendships don't just happen. Most need some care if they are to develop into that special kind where you each feel important and worthwhile. You want your thoughts and feelings to be respected and held in confidence and your friends want you to do the same.

How does a friendship get started? After all, you stutter and feel that that makes a big difference. If you've had a close friend all your life, someone you grew up with, that's great. But what if your family moved? How do you meet someone? If you stutter, you may be hesitant to make the first move. You remember from past experience that when you are trying hard not to stutter, you probably will. You worry that the way your stuttering sounds and looks will turn off potential friends and make you feel embarrassed.

It's easier to get acquainted with others if you share common interests. It's easier to put stuttering in the background if you can focus on something else. Ask yourself what you do during your free time. Is there a sport or hobby you're good at? Is there a talent you can develop? Focus on your strengths and let them outweigh your weaknesses.

To some friends, the stuttering you do makes no difference. They treat you the same whether or not you speak fluently. Your own attitude sets the tone for their reaction. If you don't appear too bothered, chances are they won't either.

But what happens if other friends look away when you stutter or answer the question before you even finish asking it? It hurts when people you have counted on for support are bothered by your stuttering. But unless you tell them, they can't really know what stuttering is like.

Do They Try to Protect You?

Do you wonder if your friends are disappointed or embarrassed when you stutter? It's easy to get that impression if they answer for you or intervene so that you can get by with talking very little. Probably they're just trying to help.

Take a closer look. Why are they trying to protect you? Do they think they are doing you a favor? Resist that kind of favor if you can. Although it may seem easier right now when they run interference for you, their protection puts off your doing what you need to do for yourself. To talk.

Suppose you're not ready to ask your friends to let you talk for yourself. You're not sure you can handle it and you're not sure how they will react when you ask them. Telling them may be taking a risk but maybe not as big a risk as you think. In the long run, it's better for you to talk and stutter–but to talk for yourself–than it is for you to keep silent and feel lousy.

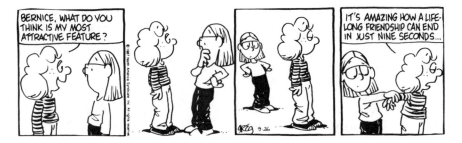

Who Orders the Cokes?

Do you chime in with 'same here' or nod in agreement even though you'd rather have something different to eat or drink? Friends are likely to understand what it's like to avoid something that is scary or embarrassing and not push you to talk for yourself. They may also be puzzled about how saying a few words can be so difficult for anyone.

You probably feel pressured to give your order quickly and think you only have one chance to do it right. This situation can be very frustrating if you're not the boss of your mouth or your head. If you are uptight about making a mistake in talking, you probably will. Worry can have a negative effect on anyone. Feeling scared affects how our bodies work. A star athlete may miss the free throw that the basketball teams needs to win the game **if** he feels pressured and **if** he lets that pressure get to him. You may miss the basket. You may stutter. But you can learn, with help from a speech pathologist, to resist pressure to speak quickly. You can learn to talk more smoothly–**if that's important enough to you.**

Do You Suffer from the 'Ma Bell Conspiracy'?

For many people who stutter, the telephone may be the situation they fear the most.

Would it surprise you to learn that some very fluent people avoid talking on the phone? They would rather communicate in person than talk to a voice somewhere out in space. Many people who stutter dislike talking on the phone until they have found better ways to cope with their speech.

That makes sense. The telephone is near the top of their list of difficult situations. It may be near the top of yours too! But it doesn't have to stay there. If you're not as fluent on the phone as you want to be, you could experiment. Find a place where what you say is more private. No one in your family is listening to you. Wait until you have lots of time and nobody is rushing you to hang up so that they can use the phone. Call people who already know you stutter some of the time and aren't bothered by it. Think about the message you want to say instead of telling yourself "careful, you might stutter." Find out what phone strategies work for you and try them out today!

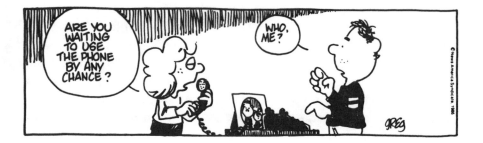

Where Do All the Friends Go?

You're at an age when people often feel lonely. It's not just you. Look at the fluent teens you know; their Saturday nights may be dead too. It's easy to think that stuttering is the culprit and get too focused on yourself.

Stuttering may contribute to the problem but not always in the way you think. If you stutter a lot, you don't talk as much as people do when they're fluent—that's obvious. As a result, you may not have developed as many conversational skills which are helpful in relationships with others. As you work on your speech, these skills will begin to come naturally.

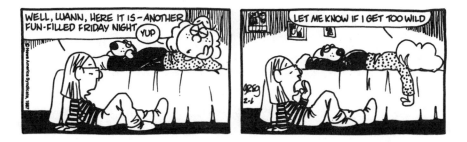

If You're In, Someone's Out.

Making fun of others—everybody does it. It separates the 'in' group from the 'out' group. If you're an "innie," you're probably not made fun of at all—not about your speech or anything else. In fact, maybe you're doing some of the teasing yourself, only it's not about speech.

Suppose you're an "outie"? Once again, this is the time for you to focus on the things you can do or know really well. As you learn how to cope with your speech, your stuttering is less likely to be a target for teasing.

If you're hassled, you can surely use a friend who cares about you. Talk to that friend about how you feel. Sharing feelings instead of keeping them inside can lessen the hurt.

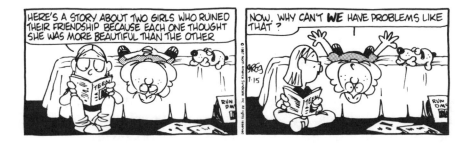

Do New People Really React to your Stuttering?

It's likely they react with surprise simply because they were not expecting you to stutter. There's no obvious sign that one person stutters and somebody else doesn't until they open their mouths to talk. Most people are curious about a behavior they haven't seen before. And they're likely to have questions such as "do you stutter because you're nervous?" Some of the mystery will be removed when you answer their questions.

Do you avoid talking to new people? You may worry how long it will be before they find out you stutter. Perhaps you think stuttering will make a bad first impression and that you will never get a second chance. Our advice is to tell them right away you do stutter sometimes. This will take a lot of the pressure off you to hide your stuttering and should make you feel better from the very start.

If you handle your stuttering in a fairly positive way, then they too will react in a more positive way. Remember that if your actions show that stuttering is no big deal to you, it probably won't be for them either.

Chapter Six

Starting To Help Yourself

Barry Guitar, Ph.D
Professor
Department of Communication Sciences and Disorders
Director, Hearst Laboratory
The University of Vermont

What can you do about your stuttering?

You can do a lot of things to improve your stuttering. Most of them are easier when you are working with a therapist. But you can do a lot of your own. This chapter will get you started.

You have probably tried things already, and many of them may not have helped much. Or, if they worked for a while, they didn't work in the long run. Like saying "uh" or "um" before saying a hard word, or saying the word silently to yourself before trying it out loud, or not taking a shower after gym class, because once that seemed to make it easier to talk. Why should **our** ideas work any better?

The authors of this book have worked with hundreds of teenagers who stutter. We have learned things which have helped a lot of teenagers who stutter. Besides which, many of us are stutterers ourselves, and we have an insider's view of what works. I can tell you from personal experience that if you can change how you feel about your stuttering, as well as change how you speak when you stutter, you can improve your stuttering so much that it may not be a bother any more.

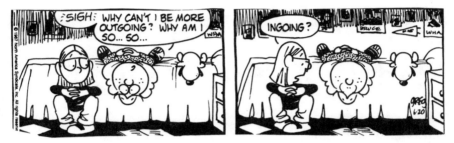

How Can You Change How You Feel About Stuttering?

One thing is for sure. The worse you feel about stuttering, the worse it gets. The more you don't want to stutter, the more you do stutter. So what can be done? How can you turn it around, so the better you feel about stuttering, the less you stutter?

How do you start? By realizing that most people aren't half as bothered by your stuttering as you are. Even if you are a severe stutterer, most people—after they get over the surprise of seeing you in the middle of a stuttering block—don't notice it as much as you think. What they notice, instead, is how bothered you are. If you seem nervous and embarassed, they are embarassed right along with you. But again, turn it around. If you could find a way to be more at ease when you stutter, they would be at ease too.

Your feelings will change and your stuttering will be less of a problem if you don't think of it as a BIG problem. Naturally, you're worried that it will screw up your life. It doesn't have to. For one thing, stuttering doesn't need to wreck your social life. Some of the sexiest people have been stutterers. Marilyn Monroe, to name one. Girls aren't usually turned off to a male stutterer unless he's so embarrassed by it that he never even squeaks. Boys usually couldn't care less whether a girl stutters or not, unless the girl lets it bother her so much she hardly ever tries to talk. And when a boy and girl get close, stuttering is not likely to be a problem, either. Speaking comes much more easily when two people know each other well.

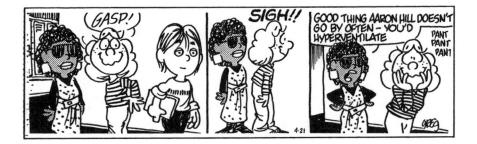

What about your job? Suppose the job you want will require a lot of talking? Many people who stutter communicate easily on their jobs. They may stutter selling cars or buying construction materials but they know their stuff and they talk anyway and their confidence carries them through the rough spots. I know of a severe stutterer who announces things over a loudspeaker at a drive-in movie as part of his job. He hardly lets his stuttering bother him at all. I have heard interviews with race car drivers and famous football players who stutter. Two of the biggest talk show hosts of all time have been stutterers. But it never seemed to interfere with their speech on camera. Movie actors, radio announcers, corporation presidents, college professors, doctors, lawyers—the world is full of people who stutter who don't let it stand in their way. Once again, your attitude about your stuttering will influence the people around you. If you treat your stuttering like it's less of a problem, so will the people around you. How do you do that?

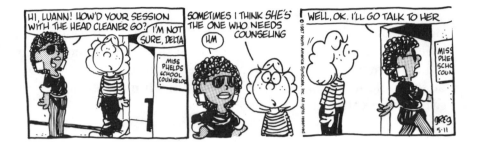

How Do You Build Confidence?

1. Remember, confidence comes slowly. You feel a little of it, then it slips away, then it comes back a little stronger.

2. You can build confidence by taking small steps and pausing to look back to see how far you've come. Fluency, like confidence comes slowly and slips back from time to time. Pick out your improvements and pat yourself on the back for them.

3. Realize that the biggest confidence builder is learning to handle failures. Trying. Falling down. Then getting back on your feet and going on. Confidence also comes when you fail and then figure out what you might do differently when you try again.

Any time you try anything new there's a chance you will fail. If you're a boy and you call a girl for a date for the first time, she may say she has to spend the weekend rearranging her sock drawer. If you're a girl and you try to talk to a cute guy, he may act like you're from another planet. You feel hurt. It may sting for a long time afterward. You feel lousy. But the reason you failed may not be because you stuttered.

If you ask someone out for a date and they say no, it may be because you took them by surprise. It may be just a matter of talking to them more and getting to know them, before they say yes. And sure, there are some people who might never go out with you. But there are plenty of fish in the sea, plenty of others to ask. The point is, you build confidence when you go ahead and try.

It hurts when you give a report in front of class and get stuck on every word. You turn beet red. Your friends snicker and jab each other. The teacher shifts around in her chair like she has ants in her pants. But if you can find the courage to keep on going, you can also find the courage to do some other positive things about your stuttering.

You can learn from a lousy experience like this. What made it so hard to talk? Did you find yourself paying more attention to your friends' snickering than to the good listeners? That's natural, but can you tune in to the good listeners in your class next time? What made it so easy to lose your concentration? Did you worry so much about stuttering that you didn't rehearse your report thoroughly enough? I've done that too. Next time wouldn't it help to prepare so well that you really know what you are going to say, so your mind is free to relax?

4. Here's another step toward confidence. Just as your feelings influence your actions, your actions can change your feelings. For example, consider how you'd stutter if you decided to act

confident when you stuttered. You'd probably be more relaxed and able to look your listener in the eye. You'd probably go ahead and say a word you wanted to, even if it meant stuttering. And when you were stuttering, you'd probably keep working on a word, without backing and filling, until you could relax your mouth and let it come out slowly.

Try it. Act the way you wish you could, and it will help to change your feelings. But remember, nobody ever became a .300 hitter overnight. Practice. Have some successes, have some failures, but learn from the part of the failure you got right. Congratulate yourself for your hard work and your good looks, and get back to work.

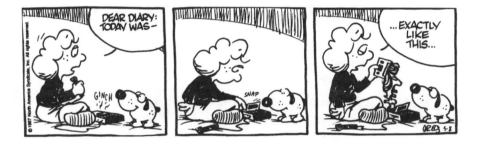

OK, You Feel A Little Better, What Can You Do About Your Stuttering?

Learn What You Do When You Stutter

Stuttering isn't some strange monster that takes over your body. Instead, stuttering is what you rush to do in your chest, throat, and mouth when you think a word might be hard to say. This is time pressure at work. The first step in changing is learning what you do when you stutter.

1. Start by studying what you do when you talk. Go somewhere alone and talk to yourself out loud. How about in the shower? Notice that you are moving your tongue and jaw and lips. Put your hand on your throat and notice that you are making sound there. Put your hand in front of your mouth and feel your breath coming out.

2. Now study what you do when you stutter. While you're still alone, pretend to stutter. Feel how you squeeze so that you are stopping yourself from talking.

3. Look for a chance to study your stuttering when you are really stuttering. Pick a time when you think you will stutter. For example, when you can see that it will be your turn to talk soon, and you think you will stutter. When your turn comes, let yourself go ahead and stutter. Don't try to stop it. This time, though, tune in to what you are doing to interrupt the flow of speech. Feel where you are squeezing. Feel if you are trying to push words out really fast. Feel if you just aren't moving some part of your speech system.

Can you do it? Can you discover what you do or don't do when you stutter? If you blow it on your first tries, don't worry. Stuttering seems to happen so fast, it's hard to notice what you're doing. Try another time. Keep trying to do this until you have a good idea of what to do to keep speech from flowing smoothly. It may take many times of thinking about what you are doing when you stutter. Remember to just let yourself stutter at first. Don't try to change it yet. When you really feel what you are doing, it will be easier to change.

Learn What You Do When You Talk More Easily

There are many different kinds of fluency. It's not that you either stutter or you don't. Sometimes you may say a hard word more easily, with only a little stuttering. Sometimes you may speak without stuttering at all. Become aware of the many ways you talk. Listen to your speech when you are talking easily. Talk to yourself alone, as you did in the shower. Feel the way your lips, and tongue, and jaw are all moving together. Feel the vibration in your throat and in your head. slow your speech down so you can pay attention to what it feels and sounds like.

Is there one thing you can tune in to most easily when you talk? The movement of your lips? Your jaw? The sound of your speech? Pick whatever is easiest and start to pay attention to that. If you can do it, you will discover you have a lot more fluency than you thought or ever noticed. Remember that fluency. Store up memories of it, like little videos in your head. You may discover you have more fluency than you thought.

Avoid Avoidances

Most stutterers keep their stuttering hot by trying not to stutter. If you're going to do something about your stuttering, you will have to do some things to cool it off.

1. Don't let yourself avoid words you might stutter on. If you dodge stuttering by substituting easier words for hard ones, you're ab-so-lutely normal, but you need to start tackling the hard words. Many words you thought were hard will become easier if you don't try to avoid them. Those that are still difficult little beggars can be handled more easily by trying to move through them in a slow and relaxed way.

2. Don't let yourself avoid speaking because you might stutter. If you find yourself not answering a question in class because you might stutter, you're just like most of us who have stuttered. But once again, this is something to change. Don't let yourself avoid talking. Talking when you are afraid is a challenge and you will sometimes fail. Big deal. Don't worry about it. But keep working on reducing the avoidances. Stuttering is like a bully inside your head. If you run from it, it comes after you. If you challenge it, it shrivels.

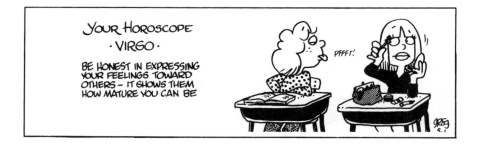

Be Open About Your Stuttering

This is the hardest, so I've saved it for nearly the last. It's hard to be open about things that bother you without feeling weird. But stuttering is one thing that gets a lot easier if you don't try to hide it.

We stutterers sometimes act like our stuttering isn't there. We try to disguise it by changing words or saying "I don't know." That almost always makes it worse. What makes it better? Talking about it. Talk to your parents. Let them read this book. Then if they ask you about it, tell them what they can do to help. Let them know if you don't want them to nag you about it. Tell them if a teacher is giving you a rough time at school about your stuttering. Talk to the therapist at school about it. If you don't have a therapist at school, talk to your parents about getting help somewhere else.

It also helps if you can make some funny comments about it. Stuttering isn't funny. but you can make it easier by making your listener feel relaxed. Then you'll feel relaxed. If you're with a friend at the Pizza Palace and you get stuck on "Pepperoni," make some offhand comment about it like, "I'm glad I got that out before they closed" or "I'm stuck on Pepperoni Pizzas" or "Easy for you to say" after the waiter repeats your order. If you can do this, your friends and other listeners will feel more at ease about your stuttering. If they feel relaxed, so will you. If **you** become less uptight, so will your mouth.

Resist Time Pressure

Notice how you tighten your mouth or your throat or your chest when you stutter? Why? Are you squeezing your muscles for exercise? No. More likely, you're struggling to get out of an uncomfortable situation. For example, say you are trying to buy something in Weasleman's Pharmacy and the word won't come out, and Mr. Weasleman is staring at you like you were an extraterrestrial. What else are you going to do but squeeze?

1. The squeezing you do when you stutter is often from trying to get the word out too fast. Have you ever seen a Chinese finger trap? It's a hollow tube the size of a lipstick. You put two fingers in, one at each end. If you try to pull your fingers out too fast, your fingers get stuck. If you pull really slowly, your fingers slide out. Like stuttering, except it's your lips or your tongue or your throat that gets stuck when you try to move too fast.

It's hard to do anything slowly. Everybody does everything quickly. How can you do anything slowly?

The only way is to work at it bit by bit. What about when your brother or sister yells to you from another room. Could you take your time when you yell back? What about when your mom or dad asks you a question? Could you take your time as you start to answer? What about when you're alone, and you're doing something like making a sandwich. Could you do it slowly? Slow motion. Now try connecting the slowness to stuttering. When you expect to stutter, can you start the word in slow motion, without squeezing? Not yet? No problem. Take your time in working on your stuttering.

2. Try stuttering slowly. Keep stuttering, but do it in slow motion. Let out a little air and a little sound. Keep it going for a moment steadily and smoothly like this: "mmmmmmmmmm..." Then SLOWLY move into the rest of the word, like "mmmmmmmmmmmaaay". You don't have to say the rest of the word slowly, but you do have to make your move out of the stutter slowly.

This might be too hard to do in most situations. Try it when you are alone, just to get the feel. If you can't do it yet when you're talking to others, put it aside until you've built up your resistance to time pressure.

Now you have a start on your own. What about getting some help? Actors have directors. Rock stars have managers. Athletes have coaches. You and a speech therapist could make a great team, working together.

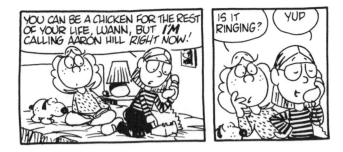

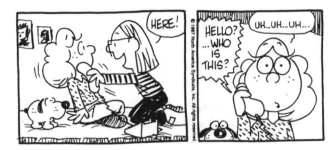

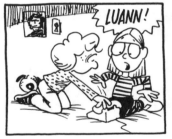

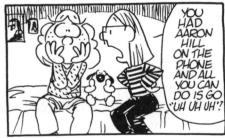

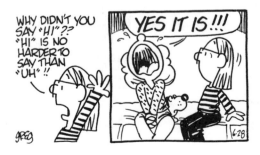

Chapter
Seven

Turning On To Therapy

William H. Perkins, Ph.D.
Professor, Communication Arts and Sciences,
Otolaryngology, and Speech Science and Technology,
Director, The Stuttering Center
University of Southern California

Why Should You Seek Help?

There are at least two answers to this question. One is that you may have to improve your speech to get what you want. This can involve getting friends, getting grades, getting parts in plays, getting jobs, getting promotions, getting respect–the list is endless. Another more important answer is if your speech bothers you enough to want to do something about it. A version of the same answer is if you want to feel more accepting of yourself as a person. These together form the best reason for seeking help because you will be doing it for yourself.

Can Therapy Do Anything for You Self-Help Can't?

Self-help has a big plus. One is that even if you're working alone, the fact that you are trying to help yourself shows your determination to not let stuttering run your life. If you bring that much determination to therapy, then your chances of success are **vastly better** than if you go to therapy hoping that the clinician will do something to you or for you that will make life easier.

What therapy can do is to help you to help yourself. A clinician can give you enough distance from your problems to get things into focus. No matter how determined you are to improve, it will be unnecessarily frustrating and slow if you don't know how to go about helping yourself. The Speech Foundation has an excellent self-help book, but it can't demonstrate some of the skills that will be useful to you.

When Should You Seek Help?

The longer you wait to start, the greater the pressure you will feel to improve your speech. As big as those pressures may seem to you now, they'll seem even bigger the closer you get to job hunting or college. Don't wait until your last semester to start. Therapy is not an overnight business. It takes time, especially for progress that will stay with you. Although you can improve in a matter of weeks, if not days, improvement can evaporate just as quickly as you learned it. All you'll have left is fog if you don't practice frequently and put what you've learned to the test on the tough words and sounds, to say nothing of the tough situations you've tried to avoid. Give yourself years, but at the very least months, if you expect therapy to work.

How Do You Cope With Aunt Buffie's Ad?

The Aunt Buffies of the world are concerned and are trying to help. If your Aunt Buffie thinks she's found help for you, remember that she's probably on your side, but also remember that she's not likely to know much about stuttering. So thank her for being interested and tell her you'll check it out. Then you are free to investigate her lead as thoroughly as you can, or want to. Who knows, she may have done you a favor. Then again maybe she unearthed a quack.

Can Therapy Cure Stuttering?

No one has found a cure for stuttering. If you hear of anyone who claims a cure—steer clear. This does not mean that some do not improve so much that they think of themselves as cured. When that happens, though, it's the exception, not the rule. If you are determined to cope with stuttering, you can improve your speech and you can improve how you feel.

Can You Believe Claims of Overnight Success?

No. Probably not, at least as far as giving you answers to whether you'll get the help you're looking for. The problem is in knowing what the claims mean. Does 98 percent success mean cured, fluency improved, feel better, or what? Many therapists could claim 100 percent success if every little improvement in fluency meant success. But that improvement would be so small as to have no meaning.

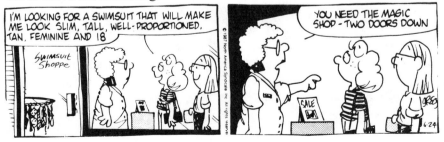

67

Good therapists don't make such claims. If a clinician hesitates to let you talk to anyone they've seen, or observe their therapy, or steer you to just certain former clients, or use testimonials from satisfied clients, or show you a slick commercial example of their success, you should be cautious. They may advertise, but the better they are the more discrete their advertising is likely to be. Good clinicians have nothing to hide. They're open for inspection.

Did You Try Therapy and It Didn't Work?

If you've had therapy before and it didn't help, you're probably convinced it won't help. Worse, you may be feeling guilty because you think it's your fault that therapy didn't work. Maybe you're also scared you'll never outgrow it. You're probably right. If you're waiting and hoping it will eventually go away, the risk is that you're waiting in vain.

Don't despair. There is hope. For one thing, the clinician you had may not have specialized in stuttering. Many therapists don't know enough about it to be of much help. But there are specialists available. Read on.

The fact is that many who are helped most were sure there was no hope. If you have doubts, but still are willing to try, talk to people who have been through different therapy programs. Good clinicians can put you in touch with most of the people they've seen. See for yourself how their speech sounds, as well as how they feel about it and themselves. Find out how much help they feel they got. Their outcome won't guarantee your outcome, but they will give you a clue as to what to expect.

Are You Afraid to Give Therapy Your Best Effort?

Nothing is quite so frightening as having to confront a moment of truth. What's scary about giving your best effort is the prospect that it might not be good enough. You might fail. If that's as far as you let yourself think, if you only look ahead as far as the possibility of failure, then fear will paralyze you. Try going beyond the failure, though, and see what happens. Let yourself think about failure in its grossest form. Turn it over in your mind. Play with it. Make it as bad as you can make it, then play each failure scenario out as far as you can take it. When you put failure in perspective, it doesn't make it pleasant but it does make it bearable. Most important, it makes it possible to give your best effort, and increases the chance of that effort succeeding.

Is 30 Minutes a Week Enough?

In the best of all possible worlds, no. Especially if you are just beginning therapy. Until you've made substantial progress, 30 minutes a week, even an hour a week, is like going to the movies and seeing nothing but previews. Momentum helps and it's tough to get it even with a couple of hours a week. Still, if you can only get an hour or so a week, progress will be slow but it is possible. Later on, when you know what you're about and are moving out on your own, brief weekly sessions can be particularly useful.

How Do You Find Help?

Before you go shopping for therapy, work out a shopping list. Do some reading about stuttering and the various therapies that have been developed for it. The Speech Foundation is a non-profit organization that specializes in help for people who stutter. They have publications containing the information you need for your shopping list.

How Do You Find a Therapist You'll Like?

Therapists help people who stutter several different ways. No single therapy or therapist is right for everyone. Finding the right therapist who can give you the help you want as well as the help you need is as difficult as finding the right girl friend or boy friend. Don't despair, though, it is possible.

The Stuttering Foundation can steer you to specialized help, but you'll have to decide if the therapist is for you. The only way you'll find out is to give whoever it is a try. First impressions aren't always right, but if you have strong objections, this therapist may just be wrong for you. If you've done your homework and prepared your shopping list (see "How do you find help?") you'll probably have a number of questions you'll want to discuss in those first sessions.

Finding the right clinician to help you isn't like finding a mechanic for your car or a surgeon for your appendix. Skill and knowledge alone aren't enough. Until you find a therapist who is both skilled and really cares about you, keep shopping.

A Personal Message

Charles Van Riper, Ph.D.
Distinguished Professor Emeritus
Western Michigan University

When I was a teenager almost seventy years ago the future sure looked bleak. I was a very severe stutterer with many long hard blockings accompanied by facial contortions and head jerks that not only provoked rejection by my listeners but also made it almost impossible for me to communicate. I'd had therapy at a stutterer's institute, gained a bit of temporary fluency, then relapsed and was worse than I'd been before. Only once had I asked a girl for a date and her answer was, "I'm not that hard up." Recitation in school was so frustrating to myself, my classmates and the teacher that I rarely said a word. Strangers, watching me try to talk, thought I was either epileptic or crazy. Those years were dark ones.

But the worst part of them was that I felt not only helpless but hopeless. How was I ever to get a job or to be able to support myself? How was I ever to get married and raise a family? I felt naked in a world full of steel knives. I thought of suicide and tried it once but failed at that too.

If a fortune teller back then had predicted that I would have a wonderful and rewarding life I would have laughed in her face, bitterly. But, despite my stuttering, or even because of it, I have such a life, and you can, too. Now eighty two years of age I can look back at those years with a sense of fulfillment. I had a fascinating job that helped me pioneer a new profession. I married a lovely woman, had three children and nine grandchildren, all of whom gave me the love I hungered for but never expected to get. I made a lot of money from the many books I wrote. I made films, TV and radio appearances; I made speeches to large audiences and gave lectures all over this country and in many foreign lands. I've had everything I wanted and more. In my old age I am content.

Surely I must have been cured of my stuttering to do all those things? No, I've stuttered all my days. I guess I'm one of those incurable stutterers. Everyone has his own personal demon and mine is stuttering. So is yours. I found that once I accepted it as a problem and learned to cope with it by not avoiding or hiding or struggling with it, my demon lost its hold on me. If I feared stuttering I talked anyway. If others rejected me because of it, well, to hell with them! I stopped fighting myself when I stuttered; I learned to stutter easily and when I did so I became fluent enough to accomplish anything I set out to do.

I've known hundreds of stutterers who managed to live equally satisfying lives despite their stuttering. Among them have been laborers, preachers, teachers, lawyers, even an auctioneer. The one characteristic they had in common was that they didn't let their stuttering prevent them from talking.

So there is hope for you too, my friend.

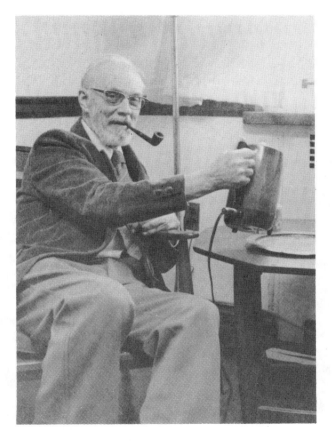

The Stuttering Foundation of America is a non-profit charitable organization dedicated to the prevention of stuttering and the improvement of treatment for stutterers. If you feel that this book has helped you and you wish to help this cause, send a tax-deductible contribution to us at P.O. Box 11749, Memphis, Tennessee 38111. Thank you.

"yearbook"

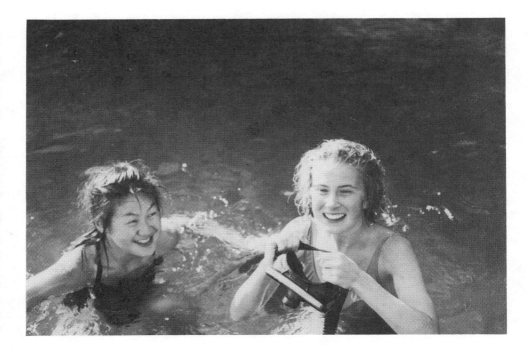

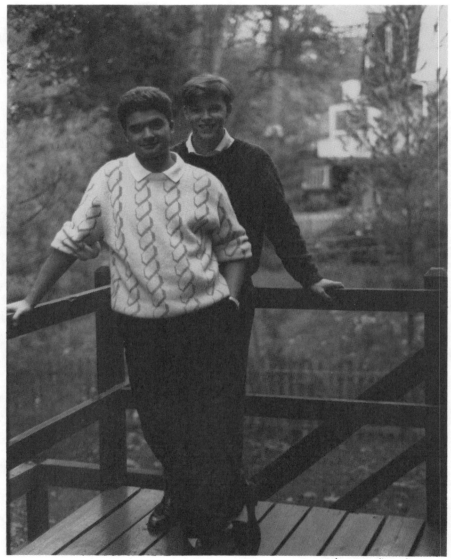

photo credit: celia gruss

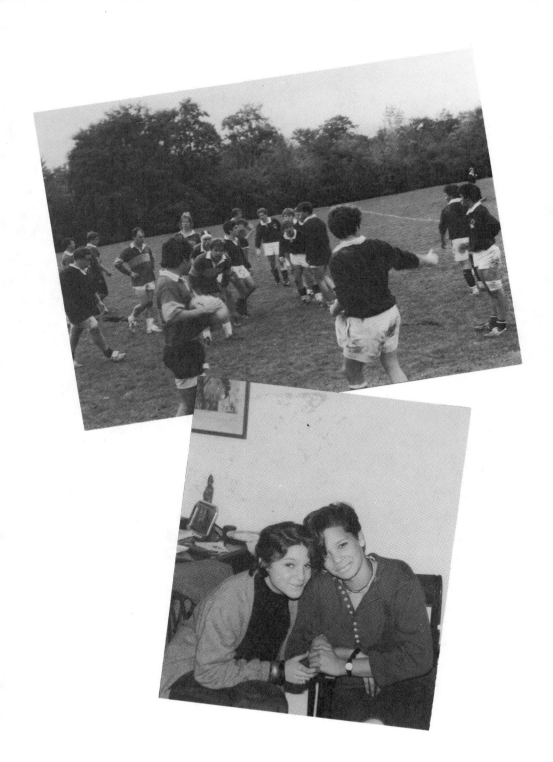

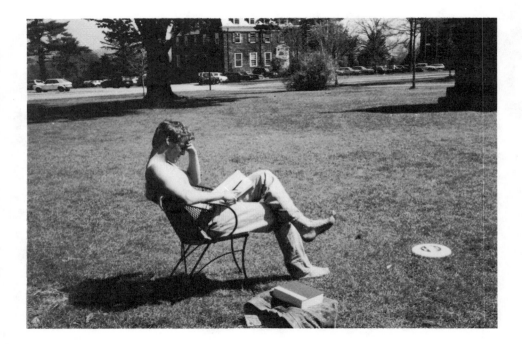

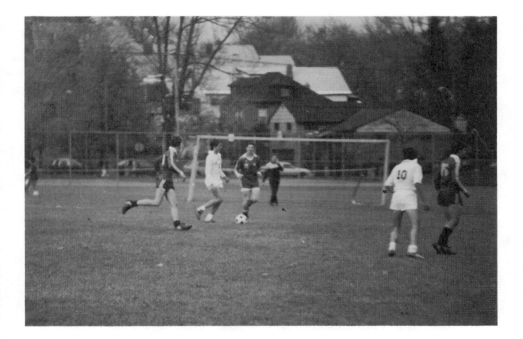

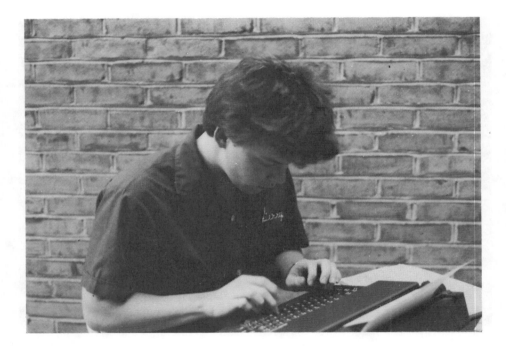